SRI JOYDIP ASHRAM

I0414708

THE YOGA OF DANCE

SRI JOYDIP

The Art of Stillness, while moving your body.

Contents

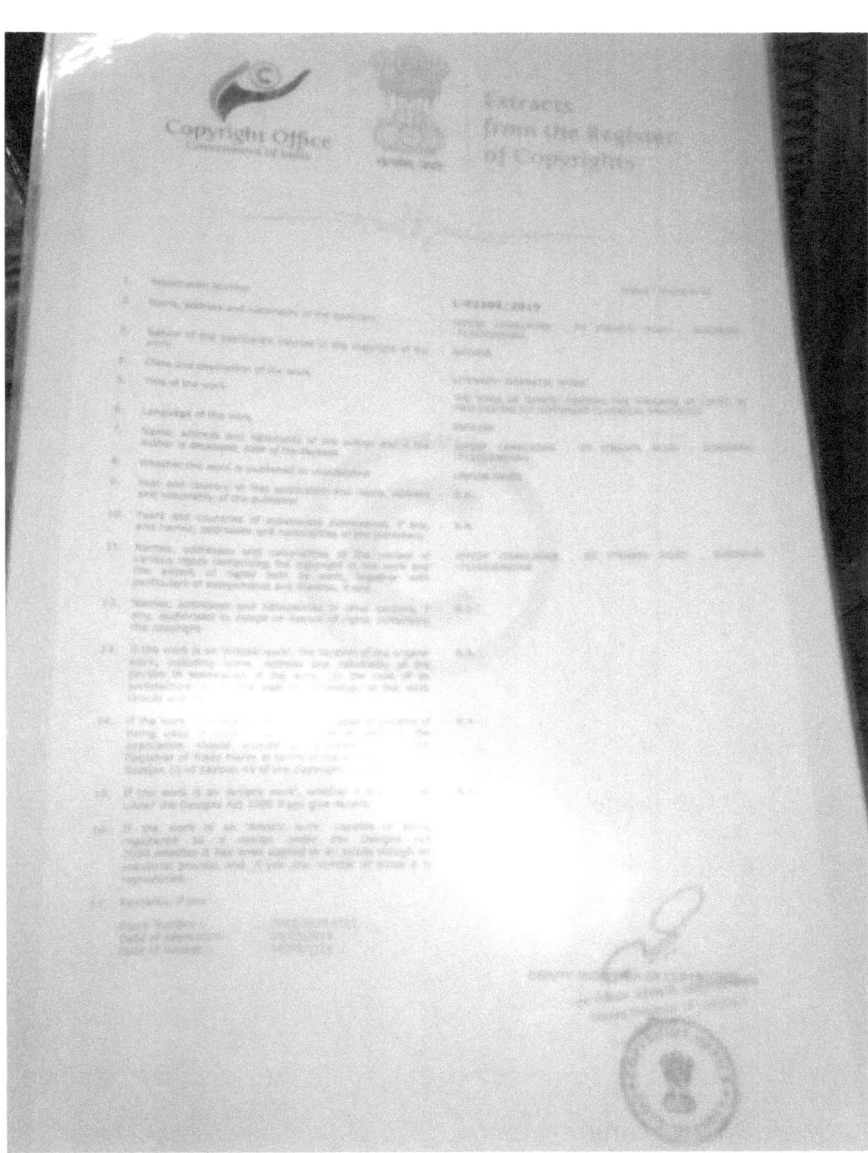

Dedication

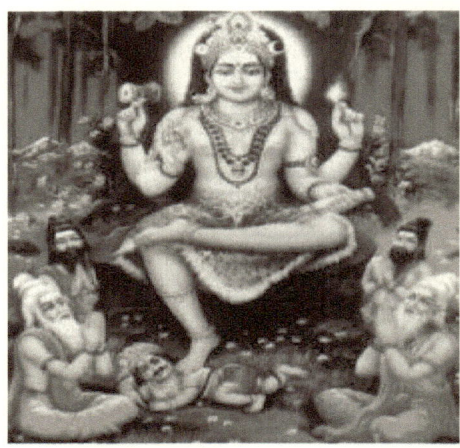

This book is dedicated to Sri Dakshinamurty, also known as 'Medha Dakshinamurty', and considered as World's first yoga teacher. He is credited for teaching yoga to the 'Saptarishis' – the seven great sages, and 'Sanakas' – the son of creator - Brahma.

While teaching yoga to Sanakas and Saptarishis, he never uttered a word. So, how did, he teach the subtle and deeper states of awareness of yoga, without using any words?

According to ancient text on Sri Dakshinamurty, he did it through silence, with displaying 'Gyan mudra'. Mudras are important hand gestures which are used both in Yoga and Dance. This phenomenon of a deity displaying mudra and communicating with his subject, was considered as purest and most artistic demonstration of yoga. It was also considered as one of the best way to demonstrate the capabilities of yoga, across the world on different time periods.

We are grateful to Sri Dakshinamurty, the first yoga teacher of the world, for blessing humanity, to travel such a long distance, crossing few centuries and yet being able to transmit the wisdom and power of yoga.

The teachings of this book, obviously is through words, which is considered, inferior to silence, to transmit the sublime and subtle experience of Yoga. That's why , I pray with all humbleness and gratitude, to Sri Dakshinamurty, and the lineage of yoga teachers, which started from him , who worked tirelessly, through centuries using yoga, for alleviating human suffering, both physical , psychological and spiritual, that this small book, may fulfil the purpose of connecting this age old tradition of alleviating human suffering, with another classical tradition of Dance.

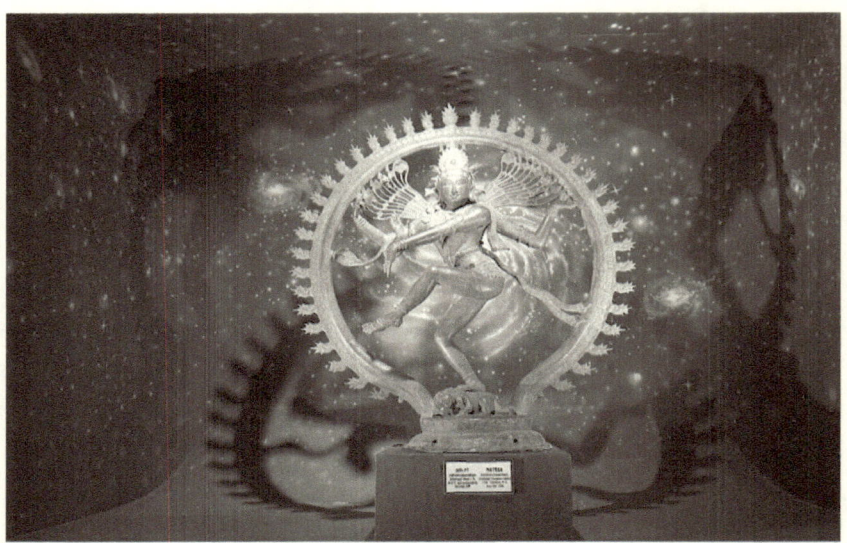

This book is also dedicated to Sri Nataraja – the Cosmic dancer, who is known as lord of Dance. This idol is taken from the famous Chidambaram Temple in South India, where the lord of dance is seen to be doing ananda tandava –The Dance of Creation.

I experience a drawing of similar type, while visiting a small temple in South India dedicated to South Indian poet Manikkavasagar. Originally hailing from Chidambaram temple, Manikkavasagar, visited Tiruvannamalai , a pilgrimage site for Shaivate sadhaks around Arunachala hill, which is considered as sacred hill , embodying qualities of Infinite consciousness, which is knows as Sivam.

It was also an important sit of Advaitic philosophy.

Manikkavasagar visited here around 8th century, and started composing Tiruvasagam his seminal work, from a small place near Adi Annamalai Temple in Tiruvannamalai . The place from where he started his poetry composition was preserved as Manikkavasagar temple, and in the floor a temple , a similar drawing exist of Lord Nataraja.

Preface

Opening up the world of Dance

It was raining heavily outside. The transition is happening between the autumn and the rainy season. I had just come back from South India. From a very boiling temperature of Tamilnadu, to an absolutely severing temperature of Bengal, my body is yet to adapt with the changes.

The rain had kept me in home. I had to discard many outdoor activities for the rain. This was a blessing in disguise, as I got some time to write a small script for a short film. The main protagonist of the film, is a dancer from Bengal, who discarded dance profession, despite her love and sincerity for the profession, facing abject poverty .

A leading Bank of India, was arranging a competition, for making short films in socially sensitive subjects. When I participated on that , I was given a subject on "Intangible heritage". So, I adapted the small script, and titled it as "A Dancer who gave up". Traditional Dance is considered as an intangible heritage, and that makes it perfectly fit for the film competition .

After completing the adaption, I contacted a Dance School in our locality. The name of the Dance school was Srijani. A teacher came to meet me from the dance school, while I was away, when I called them and told about the script . I wanted a dancer to act on the movie , as the short film is about the challenges a dancer faces, in her career in Bengal.Luckily, I also got a producer, who runs a local call centre.

Everything was going very fine as per the plan , when suddenly the producer backed up and said he cannot fund the short film . There was just two days to submit the film. And it was too short a period to find, another producer, for that same script. So, I gave up. However, while talking about this to my friend, who had been a dancer earlier, she both showed interest to act and produce the film. The film which was made in a very short budget and a short period, opened up a new world of dance to me which resulted towards a somatic transformation.

Acknowledgement

In the tenth anniversary of Sri Joydip Ashram, this little e-book was a humble effort, to present the important connection between two tradition of movement therapy. "The Yoga of Dance" in a clean, clear and concise manner. The book was based from the author's own experience of teaching Dancers, who came for help from Yoga to improve their physical agility, with different medical and psychological condition.

While going through the sessions many dancers, shared their thoughts, that they had great temporary relief, from the modern pharmacotherapy, when they faces different medical problems, but it also came with a lot of baggage of side effects.

At the same time, the author wanted to thank on behalf of Sri Joydip Ashram, all the teachers , students, volunteers, well wishers , along with beneficiaries , who have helped us to reach us, where we are today.

Yoga and Dance – The Somatic Angle

After completing the film, I found myself, more inclined to learn, more about traditional form of dance. Though the interest faded after sometime , however , in the beginning of 2019 , I attended a workshop where the dasaprana of Tala from Natya Sastra of Bharatmuni is related to Maharishi Patanjali's Asthanga Yoga.

As a long time practitioner of Yoga poses , while contemplating I found there are two aspect which is important for going deep in the practise. One is the demonstrative aspect of a Yoga pose. The other is the somatic aspect, which is how you understand and feel about your body, while you do the yoga asana. In short, what is the perception of your body, and how do you sense it is critical for healing your body.

In fact, this understanding could be quite therapeutic. (Barton, 2011) While you move from one poses to another, with a flow, observing the perception of our body and the sensations, and how it is changing, your body becomes more sacred, and connects to the Universal body. And when this connection, happens your movements become more conscious movements, and there is possibility that you can transcend the physical laws of duality .

This phenomenon is stated in Maharishi Patanjali Yoga Sutras on the section where he writes three verses on the practise of Yogic poses.

I find that similar division of somatic and demonstrative aspect, is there in many Indian dance forms ,specially the form which has origination in Tamilnadu , known popularly as Bharat Natyam. I had a student, who was a classical dancer on Bharatnatyam, though she left practising it as she grew older. While learning asanas she would frequently referenced about his learning from the Bharatnatyam teachings.

Bharatnatyam is a major genre of Indian classical dance which originated from the Natya sastra written by Bharat muni in Tamilnadu at Second Century CE.

Apart from the performance aspect, the somatic aspect where the dancer becomes more conscious about his movements and how it is evoking different sensations, in the body and the changing the way she perceives the body. That itself, could be a healing experience for her.

Yoga and Dance with Mudras – The Practical
Angle

The consciousness on the movement, can be further explored through Dance.Yoga and Dance both uses mudra or hand gestures very heavily. Hand gestures in Yoga , is a practical element of Yoga practise which helps to channelize the energy , whereas in dance it helps to communicate different aspects of artistic manifestation. (Cain Carroll)

The deities also use mudras to give certain experience of consciousness, which can be only transmitted by different forms of mudras. This hand gestures, are often used heavily in different cultural tradition of India , to transmit artistic experience , spiritual states , energy healing . As hand is a very important portion of a body, which have multiple usage, mudras are often found in multiple usage too.

Mudras also had somatic experience both in dance and Yoga. It is similar to cognitive process which helps to recognize the moving body.

Finding the Threads of Unity between Yoga and Dance

Both, Yoga and Dance can be used as a movement therapy.

Movement is called as demonstration of life. A conscious movement can sharpen the faculties and let one to observe the sensations in his body. As the self concept of the body is improved , there can be many healing experience due to the subjective dimension of body, goes through closer scrutiny. So the threads of unity between Yoga and Dance are following

Yoga	Dance	Threads of Uity
Yoga Asanas when done consciously can become Somatic practices.	Consciousness, about the different forms of movement forms creates its own form of Somatic practices.	As the observation grows the dancer can observe the self perception, which exist in her body. This awareness could be quite

		helpful on understanding the different inner aspects of bodies movement.
Mudra Practices, hand gestures are an important part to still the mind , and make it conducive for yoga.	In dance , hand gestures plays a great role to communicate what one is going through internally (expression of somatic experiences)	Here the threads of unity can come through hand gestures where in yoga the mudras helps you to deepen the practise and make the mind focussed . In dance , it helps to create most subtle and subliminal expression.

[THE YOGA OF DANCE]

A Path towards Somatic Transformation

Growing awareness about the body through yoga asana, and breathing practices, could help a yogi to connect, with the Universal body and to transcend the dualities of physical laws which we experience in day to day basis. This could happen with traditional dance form like Bharatnatyam, where the movement can be done more consciously and it could have therapeutic effect and lead to transformation of the individual's perception about his body. This kind of transformation is considered as Somatic transformation and both yoga and dance sets the path for Somatic transformation.

Rasasamadhi for Somatic Transformation

An interesting conversation on Rasasamadhi , on "Yoga of Dance finding the threads unity of two distinctly different classical practices of Bharatnatyam and Asthanga Yoga" , in Sri Joydip Ashram,Burdwan with Ramkrishna Chattopdhyay

Senior Research Fellow from Rabindra Bharati University, working on how bharatnatyam embodies the principle of ashtanga Yoga, and Founder of Bharat Kala Manjari, one of the most prominent Dance Institution in Burdwan.

The discussion was based on Sri Joydip Ashram innovative Work on "Yoga of Dance finding the threads unity of two distinctly different classical practices of Bharatnatyam and Asthanga Yoga" a separate ebook available in Amazon , referenced in the Book "Innovation@Yogaeducation:The Sri Joydip Ashram Story".

As per the Section 6(17),(18) of Sri Joydip Ashram Trust Deed specifying the objects of Sri Joydip Ashram Trust we are regularly holding such discussion with head of other education and cultural institution to create collaborative special projects education and cultural with institution having similar aim to uplift consciousness for building a meta institute that can bring social changes and help on nation building.

On the base of this discussion soon we are going to

announce our collaborative special projects between Sri Joydip Ashram and Bharat Kala Manjir for uplifting consciousness.

Understanding Rasa Samadhi

The purpose of Bharatnatyam is to achieve rasa and the purpose of asthanga yoga is to attain Samadhi . Can a Samadhi be attained while a dancer is merged into his creative expression and experiencing Rasa. Rasa is the emotional experience of Bharatnatyam and Samadhi is the ultimate step and experience and it can be found that there is an inner harmony a thread of unity which embraces the mind of dancer where he / she can attain a Samadhi while externally being involved in the act of dancing. This is where there is a meeting point between the Lord of Dance – Nataraja and the Lord of Yoga – Yogeswara and when a dancer reaches that point he/she can endure is creativity because there he receives a continous flow of inspiration which doesn't get diluted with external circumstances.

Enduring Creativity in Bharatnatyam Dance practise using Patanjali's Yoga Sutras

Bharatnatyam and Astanga Yoga are both classical practise and both of them have certain similarities and certain differences. Astanga Yoga can help to endure creativity whereas Bharatnatyam helps to demonstrate yoga and rase experience. Dancing is an phenomenon whose objective is Rasa , where is astanga yoga is an philosophy whose ultimate purpose is Samadhi. When both of them is put together it can be therapeutic , spiritual and transcending experience. Though Bharatnatyam is popularly considered as a storytelling form with lots of entertainment element , in essence it had the energies which helps one to transcend oneself and can be a very spiritual experience.

In this section we are going to explore how Bharatnatyam embodies the astanga principles of yoga. Bharatnatyam is a classical dance style from southern India and used for interpretive storytelling dance form. Astanga Yoga is based from Yoga sutra of Patanjali.

The sutras of Astanga yoga, provides an clarity on how dance movement, feet position and percussive rhythm facilitate the inner experience of Dance.

Influence of Yoga in Dance

Yoga has influenced dance teaching techniques, choreography, and performance through changes and shifts in practise, and artistic exchange through friendship , conversation, flow and collaboration. Threads of Ashtanga Yoga practise, have historically blended ,with Indian classical dance forms like Bharatnatyam , helping to communicate the inner spiritual experiences of yogis to the larger social diaspora.

Reflection on BharatNatyam

Bharatnatyam is a classical dance style from Southern India practised as an interpretive storytelling art form, that narrates vignettes and stories, from mythology , religion,history and romantic poetry. It is percussive with precise feet movements, and stamping, fluid in its body movement ,vigorous in arm movement , expressive with sophisticated hand gestures , emotional in dancers experience of the song and communicative with facial expression. The dancer dances in the synchrony with the rhythm of the music and experiences the bhava (emotions) lyrics that are sung in varying melodic patterns. The dancer utilizes the mudra (hand gestures) and abhinaya (expression) to convey his emotional experience to the audience. The non verbal interaction between the dancer , musician and audience , creates a collaborative creation of dancing experience called Rasa is the purpose of Bharatnatyam determined by Natyasastra a treatise on Indian Dramaturgy by Sage Bharata.

Reflection on Astanga Yoga

Astanga Yoga is based on the principles outlined by Yoga sutras, written by Sage Patanjali , prior to 400 CE .The Astanga prescribes eight principles that when practised leads to a union (Samadhi) of human self with the metaphysical universal being (Iswara). Bharatnatyam founds to be related to the astanga principles of Yoga , leading to dancer experience to dance , similar to Yogis experience of Samadhi which can be called as Rasa-samadhi. The practise of Astanga Yoga also helps a Bharatnatyam Dancer to harmonize his body and mind , with Universal source of energy and endure his creative energy.

Impact in Society:

Bharatnatyam & Astanga Yoga, put together can have a very positive impact on society, making it more peaceful, stress free, happy , compassionate and collaborative.

Epilogue : My Perspective on Bhartnatyam and Astangha Yoga and its impact in society.

As a writer , I create languages to express voices , feelings. To me Bharatnatyam is a language. It helps to express the feelings or bhava which the dancer receives from the music. And to articulate those feelings with movements and expression that the feeling is transmitted to the audience .

When I write a story , I get the music from my own perception , what is the way I see the world , and I had to create a literature which has to transmit that music to my readers , in a way my expression are in a word , and bharatnatyam expression is in movements on how to transmit that feelings .

It happens to be , I wrote more books on "Yoga" then I wrote on Love , politics and other issues which also create that spark me to write. Specially Asthanga yoga has been creating a lot of spark for me . One of the things , we have to learn from from Maharashi Patnajali , who is the composer of the most authentic text of asthanga yoga is brevity and universality.

Maharishi never wasted a word . Though he was brief , he was absolutely clear about what he is taking . So when he starts on uttering the word "atha yoganusana" he makes it absolutely clear that it is talking about a teaching which is a discipline.

It was not that he was the first writer on Yoga . Just before him was the mighty Sage Vyasa , and Sage Valmiki who where master story tellers. Such was the depth and outreach of there story , that we Indians after so many years have not been able to get out from the stories of Ramayana and Mahabharata.

Maharishi Patanjali , didn't wrote any stories , there was no Rama who was waiting for the explanation from Sage Vasistha , to understand the deeper truth of Yoga. There was no Arjuna , who was also guided by Sri Krishna , to understand the subtle truth of Yoga.

Maharishi Patanjali was directly speaking to his reader , instead of taking help of characters. As there was no character , there was no story which can connect it with a particular culture, his message could not be hijacked by any religion. That is the very reason , yoga become a global phenomenon.

The west completely absorbed his work . Not that he was the first writer in Yoga , but he kind of represent the earlier writers and the tradition of yoga from the 196 sutras spread around 4 chapters . Though in the medieval age it lost to other text of yoga like Bhagvad Gita , but it made a comeback at 20th century with Swami Vivekananda.

And yogasutras became classic and the foundation text of asthanga yoga.

" *Yogasutras are guide to art of Stillness, whereas Bharatnatyam is a guide to art of movement .*

Stillness, is most difficult movement, making you move, towards source of movement.

Bibliography

Barton, E. J. (2011). *Movement and Mindfulness: A Formative Evaluation of a Dance/Movement and Yoga Therapy Program with Participants Experiencing Severe Mental Illness*. American Journal of Dance Therapy.

Cain Carroll, R. C. *Mudras of India: A Comprehensive Guide to the Hand Gestures of Yoga and Dance.*

www.ingramcontent.com/pod-product-compliance
Lightning Source LLC
Chambersburg PA
CBHW020332290526
45785CB00007B/3036